THE *Skinny*
15 MINUTE MEALS
& *HIIT* WORKOUT PLAN

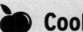 CookNation

THE SKINNY 15 MINUTE MEALS & HIIT WORKOUT PLAN
CALORIE COUNTED 15 MINUTE MEALS WITH WORKOUTS FOR A LEANER, FITTER YOU

ISBN 978-1-911219-49-1

A CIP catalogue record of this book is available from the British Library

● ●

DISCLAIMER

Some recipes may contain nuts or traces of nuts. Those suffering from any allergies associated with nuts should avoid any recipes containing nuts or nut based oils.
This information is provided and sold with the knowledge that the publisher and author do not offer any legal or other professional advice.
In the case of a need for any such expertise consult with the appropriate professional.
This book does not contain all information available on the subject, and other sources of recipes are available.

A basic level of fitness is required to perform the workouts in this book. Any health concerns should be discussed with a health professional before embarking on any of the exercises detailed.

This book has not been created to be specific to any individual's requirements. Every effort has been made to make this book as accurate as possible. However, there may be typographical and or content errors. Therefore, this book should serve only as a general guide and not as the ultimate source of subject information.

This book contains information that might be dated and is intended only to educate and entertain.

The author and publisher shall have no liability or responsibility to any person or entity regarding any loss or damage incurred, or alleged to have incurred, directly or indirectly, by the information contained in this book.

CONTENTS

DINNER

HIIT PLAN WORKOUTS

OTHER COOKNATION TITLES

INTRODUCTION

If you are time-poor but want to eat healthy, delicious, nutritious meals every day AND perform fat burning, high intensity workouts without spending hours in the gym....you can, and all in 15 minutes or less!

In our fast paced way of life, healthy, balanced and nutritious meals are often the first thing to be compromised. "I haven't got time to cook", "I'll eat on the go" or "I'll skip lunch and eat later" are just some of the excuses we all use throughout our hectic lives resulting in poor diet choices, sluggishness and weight gain.

If you are following a diet, meal choices, as well as daily exercise can become even more difficult and the added pressure of finding time to prepare food can cause you to fall at the first hurdle.

Here's the good news. If you are time-poor but want to eat healthy, delicious and nutritious meals every day AND perform fat burning, high intensity workouts without spending hours in the gym....you can, and all in 15 minutes or less! **The Skinny 15 Minute Meals & HIIT Workout Plan** brings over 60 breakfast, lunch and dinner recipes to the table in 15 minutes or less and all below 300, 400 or 500 calories each. Plus our high intensity sessions incorporate over 25 illustrated exercises to perform at home, with no equipment in 15 minutes.

If you think you haven't got time to cook and exercise...think again. You could be eating delicious, skinny, fat burning meals and training your core every day in just 15 minutes.

The majority of recipes serve one and are big on flavour and nutrition – no compromises.

THE SECRET TO 15 MINUTE MEALS

Preparing and cooking meals in 15 minutes or less requires a little help from modern convenience stores in the shape of some carefully selected pre-prepared products. Slashing prep times is how you can make 15 minutes meals in a flash.

By altering your shopping habits a little, your fridge and store cupboard can be regularly stocked with super-fast pre-prepared ingredients that make meals simple – less time, less fuss, less washing up! We're not talking highly processed fast food but instead, freshly prepared ingredients that will save you the time chopping, washing, peeling, grating and all the other laborious tasks that add minutes to your kitchen prep.

To follow is a list of some of the most common pre-prepared smart buys used in our recipes that will slash time off your cooking. This is not however a comprehensive shopping list, so check which recipes you plan to follow and shop accordingly.

- Jar crushed chilli flakes
- Bags pre sliced/chopped onions
- Bags pre sliced/chopped red onions
- Bags prepared carrot batons
- Bags washed, sliced mushrooms
- Bags washed rocket, spinach and mixed salad leaves
- Bags prepared shredded kale & spring greens
- Packets trimmed asparagus tips
- Packets trimmed green beans
- Packets shelled fresh peas
- Pre-grated low fat cheddar cheese
- Pre-grated Parmesan cheese
- Packets straight-to-wok noodles
- Packets ready-to-go microwaveable rice
- Bottle of lime juice
- Bottle of lemon juice
- Jar sundried tomatoes in oil
- Curry powder
- Pre-cooked chicken breast

Remember that pre-prepared just means someone has already done some of the work for you. The ingredients we suggest are still nutritious, fresh and full of flavour – no compromises on taste or goodness. Adding these items may add a few extra pennies to your weekly shopping budget but the time you'll save in the kitchen will be worth it. Plus you'll be eating great-tasting, healthy, calorie counted meals every day…in just 15 minutes.

You could of course prepare many of these ingredients yourself when you have more time and have them ready in the fridge to use when preparing your 15 minute meals.

PREPARATION & COOKING TIMES
All the recipes should take no longer than 15 minutes to prepare and cook. This is based on making full use of our suggestions for some pre-prepared ingredients. If you prefer to prepare your ingredients from scratch then obviously allow longer prep time.

All meat should be trimmed of visible fat and the skin removed.

NUTRITION
All of the recipes in this collection are balanced low calorie meals which should keep you feeling full. It is important to balance your food between proteins, good carbs, good fats, dairy, fruit and vegetables.

Protein. Keeps you feeling full and is also essential for building body tissue. Good protein sources come from meat, fish and eggs.

Carbohydrates. Not all carbs are good and generally they are high in calories, which makes them difficult to include in a calorie limiting diet. However carbs are a good source of energy for your body as they are converted more easily into glucose (sugar) providing energy. Try to eat 'good carbs' which are high in fibre and nutrients e.g. whole fruits and veg, nuts, seeds, whole grain cereals, beans and legumes.

Good Fats. A small amount of fat is an essential part of a healthy, balanced diet. Fat is a source of essential fatty acids such as omega-3 – "essential" because the body can't make them itself. Fat helps the body absorb vitamins A, D and E. Good fats can be found in olive oil, rapeseed oil, avocados, almond nuts and oily fish such as sardines, salmon and tuna.

Dairy. Dairy products provide you with vitamins and minerals. Cheeses can be very high in calories but other products such as low fat Greek yoghurt, crème fraiche and skimmed milk are all good.

Fruit & Vegetables. Eat your five a day. There is never a better time to fill your 5 a day quota. Not only are fruit and veg very healthy, they also fill up your plate and are ideal snacks when you are feeling hungry.

PORTION SIZES

If your goal is weight loss, the size of the portion that you put on your plate will significantly affect your weight loss efforts. Filling your plate with over-sized portions will obviously increase your calorie intake and hamper your dieting efforts.

It's important with all meals that you use a correct sized portion, which generally is the size of your clenched fist. This applies to any side dishes of vegetables and carbs too.

The portion sizes in our 15 Minute Meal recipes are the correct size for the average adult.

THE HIIT PLAN WORKOUTS

If you are new to regular exercise or haven't been active for some time then firstly congratulations on making a positive step to getting back into shape! Exercise is a great way to improve not just your body but also your mind. Not only can regular physical activity help prevent illness it can also bring clarity and focus to your everyday life. It can help you lose weight, get trim and keep you feeling better. There are many benefits to reap from regular exercise.

Before starting on our HiiT workouts it is important to evaluate your basic level of fitness. If you have any major health concerns such as those listed below we recommend first seeking a health professionals advice.

- Heart disease
- Asthma or lung disease
- Type 1 or type 2 diabetes
- Kidney disease
- Arthritis

- Pain or discomfort in your chest
- Back pain
- Dizziness or lightheadedness
- Shortness of breath
- Ankle swelling

- Rapid heartbeat
- Smoker
- Overweight
- High blood pressure
- High Cholesterol

HiiT, or high-intensity interval training, is a new kind of training program which concentrates on you giving your maximum effort through fast, intense bursts of exercise, followed by short recovery periods. It is quick and convenient and does not require equipment so you can do it anywhere, anytime.

These predominantly cardio exercises are designed to get your heart rate up, which in turn burns more fat in less time by increasing the body's need for oxygen during the effort. This creates an oxygen shortage, causing your body to ask for more oxygen during recovery. Often referred to as Excess Post-Exercise Oxygen

Consumption (EPOC) this is the reason why intense exercise helps burn more fat and calories than traditional aerobic/cardio workouts.

Put simply regular HiiT workouts will help you increase your metabolism, reduce body fat and build lean muscle. In order to do this effectively our HiiT workouts should be combined with a healthy nutritional lifestyle, which is why the calorie counted 15 minute recipes in this book are the perfect partner. Physical and indeed everyday activities require energy to perform so we recommend a balanced diet of carbohydrates, protein and fat. Using a fitness tracker such as MyFitnessPal will help you achieve your daily nutritional needs.

Prior to performing any physical activity make sure you warm up first with some gentle stretching and exercises such as jogging on the spot and jumping jacks (see workouts from page 76).
We have compiled 4 high intensity interval training workouts to perform each week (see page 73). To begin with ease yourself into these exercises especially if it has been some time since you have engaged in any cardio based training. As you progress and feel more comfortable with the routines you can increase intensity.

You should aim to do all 4 workouts within a 7 day period (1 per day) using the remaining 3 days to rest. Try to alternate where possible between training and rest days. Rest days are important as they give your body time to recover and repair - don't be tempted to skip them. Each workout lasts for approximately 15 minutes and a simple explanation with diagrams of how to correctly perform each exercise is provided.

Over time conditioning routines (HiiT) will help to make you lean in conjunction with a healthy balanced diet. They take work, time and dedication so be sure to stick at them and increase the intensity as the weeks go by.

As you progress you can, if you wish, start to introduce some basic weights (such as light dumbbells) into some of the exercises such as squats, lunges and standing mountain climbers. Taking just 15 mins out of your day to keep fit will set you on a lifelong path to a healthier, leaner and happier you.

WORKOUT TIPS

- Warm up and cool down before and after each workout
- Have a bottle of water to drink from between sets
- Remember to breathe through each exercise
- Keep your core tight & give maximum effort
- Focus on maintaining correct posture & form for each exercise

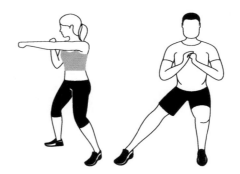

ABOUT 🍎 CookNation

CookNation is the leading publisher of innovative and practical recipe books for the modern, health conscious cook. CookNation titles bring together delicious, easy and practical recipes with their unique approach - easy and delicious, no-nonsense recipes - making cooking for diets and healthy eating fast, simple and fun.

With a range of #1 best-selling titles - from the innovative 'Skinny' calorie-counted series, to the 5:2 Diet Recipes collection - CookNation recipe books prove that 'Diet' can still mean 'Delicious'!

THE *Skinny* 15 MINUTE MEALS & *HIIT* WORKOUT PLAN

BREAKFAST

FETA OMELETTE

330 calories per serving

Ingredients

- 2 large free-range eggs
- 50g/5oz feta cheese, crumbled
- 1 tsp olive oil
- 1 tbsp freshly chopped chives
- 50g/2oz watercress
- Salt & pepper to taste

Method

1 Lightly beat the eggs with a fork. Season well and add the crumbled feta cheese and chives.

2 Gently heat the oil in a small frying pan and add the omelette mixture. Tilt the pan to ensure the mixture is evenly spread over the base.

3 Cook on a low to medium heat and, when the eggs are set underneath, fold the omelette in half and continue to cook for a further 2 minutes.

4 Serve with the watercress sprinkled all over the top.

CHEFS NOTE

Check the eggs are set underneath by lifting with a fork before folding the omelette in half.

AVOCADO & STRAWBERRY SALAD

310 calories per serving

Ingredients

- ½ ripe avocado, peeled, stoned & cubed
- 75g/3oz strawberries, sliced
- ½ tsp paprika
- 1 shallot, finely chopped
- 2 tsp lime juice
- 1 tbsp freshly chopped coriander
- 125g/4oz watercress or rocket leaves
- Salt & pepper to taste

Method

1 Combine the cubed avocado, strawberries, paprika, shallots, lime & coriander together.

2 Allow to sit for a few minutes to let the flavour infuse.

3 Pile onto a bed of watercress or rocket leaves, season & serve.

CHEFS NOTE
Stone the avocado by cutting in half (you'll need to work around the centre stone). When halved, dig the point of the knife into the stone to lever it out, then use a large spoon to scoop each half of the avocado out in one piece.

SCRAMBLED QUINOA OMELETTE

470 calories per serving

Ingredients

- 2 tsp olive oil
- ¼ red onion, sliced
- 1 yellow or orange pepper, deseeded & sliced
- ½ tsp each turmeric & paprika
- 50g/2oz cooked quinoa (cooked weight)
- 2 large free-range eggs
- Salt & pepper to taste
- 1 tbsp chopped flat leaf parsley

Method

1 Gently heat the olive oil in a frying pan and sauté the onions and pepper for a few minutes until softened.

2 Add the dried spices to the pan and stir. Cook for a minute or two longer before adding the eggs and quinoa to the pan.

3 Increase the heat, add seasoning and cook until the eggs are scrambled.

4 Check the seasoning & serve immediately. Garnish with chopped parsley.

CHEFS NOTE
You could also serve this as a lunchtime meal with a crunchy green salad.

PARMESAN & ROASTED PEPPER FRITTATA

362 calories per serving

Ingredients

- 1 tsp olive oil
- 2 shallots, chopped
- 250g/9oz roasted peppers, drained & chopped
- 3 large free-range eggs

- 1 tbsp grated Parmesan cheese
- 2 sundried tomatoes, finely chopped
- 2 tbsp freshly chopped flat leaf parsley
- Salt & pepper to taste

Method

1 Heat the oil in a frying pan and gently sauté the shallots and peppers for a few minutes until softened. Add the peppers and continue to cook for 2-3 minutes longer.

2 Break the eggs into a bowl and combine with the Parmesan cheese. Tip the sautéed onions and peppers into the bowl along with the sundried tomatoes. Mix well and return the egg mixture to the pan, tilting to ensure the mixture covers the base evenly.

3 Cover the pan, reduce the heat and leave to cook for a few minutes. Flip the frittata over and cook the other side until the eggs set and the vegetables are tender.

4 Cut into wedges and serve with chopped parsley sprinkled over the top.

CHEFS NOTE
To keep things really simple use jars of precooked roasted peppers for this recipe.

POACHED EGG & MUSHROOM TOWER

375 calories per serving

Ingredients

- 1 tbsp soft cheese
- 2 tsp freshly chopped chives
- ½ garlic cloves, crushed
- 1 large flat mushroom

- 1 large free-range egg
- ½ avocado, stoned and sliced
- 1 handful rocket leaves
- Salt & pepper to taste

Method

1 Preheat the oven grill.

2 Mix the soft cheese, chives & garlic together and spread evenly on the underside of the mushroom. Season well and place, underside up, under the grill for 5-7 minutes or until the mushroom is cooked through.

3 Meanwhile fill a frying pan with boiling water and break the egg into the gently simmering pan to poach while the mushroom cooks.

4 Put the mushroom on the plate. Arrange the rocket over the top. Add the poached egg and pile the avocado slices on top.

CHEFS NOTE
Serve seasoned with plenty of black pepper over the top.

BALSAMIC GARLIC & ROSEMARY TOMATOES

220 calories per serving

Ingredients

- 3 large beef tomatoes, quartered
- 1 garlic clove, crushed
- ½ tsp dried rosemary
- 2 tsp olive oil
- 2 tsp balsamic vinegar
- 1 red onion, sliced
- 1 small ciabatta roll
- Salt & pepper to taste

Method

1 Combine together the crushed garlic, rosemary, olive oil & balsamic vinegar and gently heat in a frying pan.

2 Season the tomatoes and sauté in the frying pan along with the onions for 8-10 minutes or until the tomatoes are softened and cooked through.

3 Cut the ciabatta roll in half and lightly toast. Pile the balsamic onions and tomatoes on top of the ciabatta halves and serve.

CHEFS NOTE
You could use any type of tomato you prefer for this recipe.

MUSTARD MUSHROOMS ON GRANARY

205 calories per serving

Ingredients

- 1 tsp olive oil
- 1 garlic cloves, crushed
- ½ onion, sliced
- 150g/5oz mushrooms, sliced
- 2 tsp Dijon mustard
- 60ml/¼ cup low fat crème fraiche
- 1 piece granary bread, lightly toasted
- 2 tsp freshly chopped flat leaf parsley
- Salt & pepper to taste

Method

1 Gently sauté the onions and garlic in the olive oil for a few minutes. Add the mushrooms and continue cooking for 8-10 minutes or until the mushrooms are soft and cooked through.

2 Stir through the mustard and crème fraiche, combine well and warm through.

3 Pile the creamy mushrooms and onions onto the granary toast and sprinkle with chopped parsley.

4 Season and serve.

CHEFS NOTE
You could substitute English mustard in this recipe but it will be a lot 'hotter'!

CAJUN SPINACH EGGS

210 calories per serving

Ingredients

- 1 red pepper, deseeded & sliced
- 1 tsp paprika
- ½ tsp each chilli powder, cumin, coriander & salt
- 2 large free-range eggs
- 1 tsp olive oil
- 75g/3oz spinach leaves
- Salt & pepper to taste

Method

1 Break the eggs into a bowl, add the dried spices & salt and lightly beat with a fork.

2 Gently heat the oil in a frying pan and add the peppers.

3 Sauté for a few minutes until they begin to soften.

4 Add the spinach and allow to wilt for a minute or two. Pour in the beaten eggs and move around the pan until the eggs begin to scramble. As soon as they start to set remove from the heat and serve with lots of black pepper.

CHEFS NOTE
You can use a ready made Cajun mix if you have one to hand.

BERRY SMOOTHIE

200 calories per serving

Ingredients

- 50g/2oz blueberries
- 50g/2oz strawberries
- 1 ripe banana
- 120ml/½ cup fat free Greek yogurt
- 1 tsp honey

Method

1 Remove the strawberry stalks and peel the banana.

2 Blend all the ingredients together. Check the sweetness of the smoothie and add a little water or ice if you want to alter the consistency.

3 Pour into a glass and serve immediately.

CHEFS NOTE

This is a really fast early morning pick-me-up. You could also add some brazil nuts to the recipe when you blend for a slightly different texture.

BLUE CHEESE OMELETTE

370 calories per serving

Ingredients

- 2 large free-range eggs
- 40g/1½oz stilton cheese, crumbled
- 1 tsp olive oil

- 50g/2oz watercress
- Salt & pepper to taste

Method

1 Lightly beat the eggs with a fork. Season well and add the crumbled blue cheese.

2 Gently heat the oil in a small frying pan and add the omelette mixture. Tilt the pan to ensure the mixture is evenly spread over the base.

3 Cook on a low to medium heat and, when the eggs are set underneath, fold the omelette in half and continue to cook for a further 2 minutes.

4 Serve with the watercress sprinkled all over the top.

CHEFS NOTE
Check the eggs are set underneath by lifting with a fork before folding the omelette in half.

THE *Skinny*
15 MINUTE MEALS
& *HIIT* WORKOUT PLAN

LUNCH

PENNE, PEAS & BEANS

375 calories per serving

Ingredients

- 50g/2oz baby broad beans
- 75g/3oz wholewheat penne
- 1 tsp olive oil
- 1 garlic clove, crushed

- 75g/3oz fresh peas
- 60ml/¼ cup low fat crème fraiche
- 1 tsp freshly chopped mint
- Salt & pepper to taste

Method

1 Blanch the broad beans and remove the skins.

2 Cook the penne in a pan of salted boiling water until tender.

3 Meanwhile gently heat the olive oil in a high-sided frying pan and sauté the blanched broad beans, garlic & peas whilst the pasta cooks. When the peas and beans are cooked through stir in the crème fraiche and mint.

4 Drain the cooked penne and add to the pan.

5 Toss well, season & serve with lots of freshly ground black pepper.

CHEFS NOTE

To blanch broad beans: plunge in unsalted boiling water and cook for 3-4 minutes until tender. Drain and cover with cold water before sliding off their skins.

FRESH ASPARAGUS & WATERCRESS SOUP

180 calories per serving

Ingredients

- 125g/4oz potatoes, finely chopped
- 1 tbsp olive oil
- 2 garlic cloves, crushed
- 1 tsp dried thyme
- 1 onion, sliced
- 1lt/4 cups vegetable stock/broth
- 400g/14oz asparagus tips
- 150g/5oz watercress
- Salt & pepper to taste

Method

1 Add all the ingredients, except the watercress, to a saucepan. Bring to the boil and simmer for 5-7 minutes, or until the potatoes are tender.

2 Roughly blend the soup with just a couple of pulses in the food processor.

3 Stir through the watercress, check the seasoning and serve immediately.

CHEFS NOTE

This soup serves 4 and can be stored in the fridge or freezer. You could use rocket or spinach rather than watercress if you wish.

AVOCADO & PRAWN COCKTAIL

390 calories per serving

Ingredients

- 1 tbsp low fat mayonnaise
- 1 tbsp low fat crème fraiche
- 1 tsp tomato ketchup
- 1 dash tobasco sauce
- 1 tsp lemon juice
- 1 tsp freshly chopped chives
- 150g/5oz cooked & peeled prawns
- ½ Romaine lettuce, shredded
- ½ ripe avocado peeled, stoned & diced
- ¼ cucumber, diced
- Pinch cayenne pepper
- Salt & pepper to taste

Method

1 Mix together the mayonnaise, crème fraiche, ketchup, tobasco sauce, lemon juice, chives & prawns until everything is really well combined.

2 In a separate bowl gently combine the shredded lettuce, avocado & cucumber to make a salad.

3 Add the salad to the plate and pile the dressed prawns on top

4 Sprinkle with cayenne pepper and serve.

CHEFS NOTE
Use paprika rather than cayenne pepper if you don't want the 'heat'.

BROCCOLI & CAULIFLOWER SOUP

190 calories per serving

Ingredients

- 200g/7oz cauliflower florets, chopped
- 200g/7oz broccoli florets, chopped
- 75g/3oz potatoes, peeled & chopped
- 1 onion, chopped
- 1 tsp ground coriander
- 1lt/4 cups vegetable stock/broth
- 250ml/1 cup semi skimmed milk
- Salt & pepper to taste

Method

1 Add all the ingredients, except the milk, to the saucepan.

2 Bring to the boil and leave to simmer for 10-12 minutes or until the vegetables are tender.

3 Blend to a smooth consistency, add the milk, and heat through for a minute or two. Check the seasoning and serve.

CHEFS NOTE
This soup serves 4 and can be stored in the fridge or freezer.

PRAWN & PAPRIKA RICE

390 calories per serving

Ingredients

- 1 tsp olive oil
- 1 garlic clove, crushed
- ½ onion, sliced
- 1 red pepper, deseeded & sliced
- 100g/3½oz cherry tomatoes, chopped
- 125g/4oz wholemeal microwavable rice
- 1 tsp paprika
- 150g/5oz peeled raw prawns
- Salt & pepper to taste

Method

1 Heat the olive oil in a frying pan and gently sauté the garlic, onions, peppers & tomatoes for 10 minutes or until everything is softened and forms a combined base.

2 Add the prawns, paprika & rice to the frying pan and cook until piping hot and cooked through.

3 Toss well. Season and serve.

CHEFS NOTE
Add a dash of water to the pan during cooking if it needs loosening up.

BALSAMIC TUNA & ZUCCHINI

370 calories per serving

Ingredients

- 2 medium courgettes/zucchinis, diced
- ½ red onion, finely chopped
- 3 tsp olive oil
- 1 fresh tuna steaks, weighing 150g/5oz
- 1 tbsp balsamic vinegar
- 75g/3oz rocket & watercress leaves
- Salt & pepper to taste

Method

1 Gently sauté the courgettes and red onion in 2 teaspoons of the olive oil for a few minutes until softened.

2 Season the tuna. Put a frying pan on a high heat with the rest of the olive oil and balsamic vinegar.

3 Place the tuna in the pan and cook for 2 minutes each side. Remove the tuna from the pan and serve with the watercress and courgette side dish.

CHEFS NOTE
Two minutes of cooking each side should leave the tuna rare in the centre. Reduce or increase cooking time depending on your preference.

FETA, PEPPERS & FILLET

495
calories per
serving

Ingredients

- 150g/5oz fillet steak
- 2 tsp olive oil
- ½ onion, sliced
- ½ garlic clove, crushed
- 1 red or yellow pepper, deseeded & sliced
- ½ tsp paprika
- 100g/3½oz cherry tomatoes
- 1 baby gem lettuce
- 50g/2oz feta cheese, crumbled
- Salt & pepper to taste

Method

1 Lightly brush the steak with a little of the olive oil. Season and put a frying pan on a high heat.

2 In another pan gently sauté the peppers, paprika, onions & garlic in the rest of the olive oil for 5-7 minutes or until tender.

3 Place the steak in the smoking hot dry pan and cook for 2 minutes each side, or to your liking. Leave to rest for 3 minutes and then finely slice.

4 Halve the tomatoes & shred the lettuce. Place in a bowl, add the sliced peppers, crumble the feta cheese, combine well and then tip into a shallow bowl.

5 Place the sliced steak on top. Season and serve.

CHEFS NOTE
Fillet steak can be expensive so feel free to use whichever cut is within your budget.

BROWN RICE & CHICKEN STIR-FRY

400 calories per serving

Ingredients

- 125g/4oz skinless chicken breast, sliced
- 100g/3½oz tenderstem broccoli
- 125g/4oz wholemeal microwavable rice
- 1 tsp olive oil
- 1 garlic clove, crushed
- ½ onion, chopped

- 2 tsp soy sauce
- 60ml/ ¼ cup chicken stock/broth
- 1 tsp fish sauce
- 200g/7oz spinach leaves, chopped
- 1 fresh lime wedge
- Salt & pepper to taste

Method

1 Season the chicken and roughly chop the broccoli.

2 Heat the olive oil in a frying pan and gently sauté the garlic and onions for a few minutes.

3 Add the chicken & chopped broccoli to the pan along with the soy sauce, chicken stock & fish sauce. Stir-fry for 8-10 minutes until the chicken is cooked through.

4 Add the rice to the pan along with the spinach. Combine for a minute or two, pile into a bowl with the lime wedge on the side. Check the seasoning and serve.

CHEFS NOTE

Sugar snap peas make a good addition to this dish.

SPICY LAMB & CARROT BURGER

SERVES 1

380 calories per serving

Ingredients

- 125g/4oz lean lamb mince
- 1 carrot, peeled & grated
- 2 tsp fresh breadcrumbs
- 1 small free-range egg
- ½ garlic clove, crushed
- ½ tsp English mustard
- Pinch of cumin
- 1 large plum tomatoes, sliced
- A few sprigs of watercress
- 1 wholemeal bread roll
- Low cal cooking oil spray
- Salt & pepper to taste

Method

1 Preheat the grill.

2 Put the lamb mince, carrots, breadcrumbs, eggs, garlic, mustard & cumin in a food processor and pulse for a few seconds to combine.

3 Season well and shape into a burger patty. Spray with a little low cal oil and place under the grill to cook for 5-6 minutes each side or until cooked through.

4 Split open the roll and when the burger is cooked through place inside the roll.

5 Lay the sliced tomatoes on top of the burger along with the watercress.

6 Season and serve.

CHEFS NOTE

This is great served with ketchup and/or a dollop of fat free Greek yogurt.

COURGETTE SPAGHETTI, TOMATOES & OLIVES

230 calories per serving

Ingredients

- 1 large courgette/zucchini
- 125g/4oz ripe cherry tomatoes
- 1 tbsp balsamic vinegar
- 8 pitted black olives, halved
- 1 tbsp olive oil

- 1 garlic clove, crushed
- ½ onion, sliced
- 1 tbsp freshly chopped basil
- Salt & pepper to taste

Method

1 First spiralize the courgette into thin spaghetti noodles.

2 Dice the ripe tomatoes and place in a bowl with the balsamic vinegar and some seasoning.

3 Heat the olive oil in a high-sided frying pan and gently sauté the garlic, onions, tomatoes and olives for a few minutes.

4 Add the courgette spaghetti and increase the heat. Stir fry for 2-3 minutes. Toss well, sprinkle with freshly chopped basil, season & serve.

CHEFS NOTE
You will need a Spiralizer for this dish if you don't have one pre-prepared shredded vegetables are now available in most supermarkets.

FRESH PEA & PRAWN NOODLES

360
calories per serving

Ingredients

- 1 tsp olive oil
- 1 garlic clove, crushed
- 1 tsp freshly grated ginger
- Pinch of crushed chilli flakes
- 150g/5oz shelled, raw king prawns
- ½ onion, sliced
- ½ red pepper, deseeded & sliced

- 2 tbsp soy sauce
- 2 tsp Thai fish sauce
- 100g/3½oz fresh peas
- 100g/3 ½oz straight to wok wholemeal noodles
- Lemon wedge to serve
- Salt & pepper to taste

Method

1 Heat the olive oil in a frying pan and gently sauté the garlic and ginger for a minute. Add the chilli flakes, prawns, onions, peppers, soy sauce, fish sauce & fresh peas and cook for 8-10 minutes or until the peppers soften and the prawns pink up.

2 Add the noodles and combine for 3-4 minutes or until the noodles are piping hot and the prawns are cooked through.

3 Season and serve with a lemon wedge.

CHEFS NOTE

This simple stir-fry works equally well with sliced chicken breast.

BROCCOLI & CHICKEN STIR-FRY

370 calories per serving

Ingredients

- 125g/4oz skinless chicken breast, sliced
- 125g/4oz tenderstem broccoli
- 1 tsp olive oil
- 1 garlic clove, crushed
- ½ onion, chopped

- 2 tsp soy sauce
- 2 tbsp chicken stock
- 75g/3oz spinach leaves, chopped
- 125g/4oz wholemeal microwavable rice
- Salt & pepper to taste

Method

1 Season the chicken and roughly chop the broccoli.

2 Heat the olive oil in a frying pan and gently sauté the garlic and onions for a few minutes.

3 Add the chicken & chopped broccoli to the pan along with the soy sauce and chicken stock. Stir-fry for 8-10 minutes until the chicken is cooked through.

4 Add the rice and stock to the pan along with the spinach.

5 Combine for a minute or two, check the seasoning and serve.

CHEFS NOTE
Microwavable rice is also suitable for stir frying as it's already cooked and just needs warming through.

CORIANDER CHICKEN & RICE

390
calories per serving

Ingredients

- 125g/4oz wholemeal microwavable rice
- 2 tsp coriander seeds
- 1 tsp fenugreek seeds
- 2 tsp olive oil
- 1 garlic clove, crushed
- ½ red chilli, deseeded & finely chopped
- 125g/4oz skinless chicken breast, sliced
- 2 tsp soy sauce
- 1 large free-range egg
- Salt & pepper to taste

Method

1 Bash the coriander and fenugreek seeds with a pestle and mortar.

2 Heat the olive oil in a frying pan and gently sauté the garlic for a minute along with the bashed seeds.

3 Add the chilli, chicken & soy sauce and cook for 5-10 minutes or until the chicken is cooked through.

4 Add the rice to the pan along with the egg. Increase the heat, stir-fry for 3-4 minutes.

5 Season & serve.

CHEFS NOTE
Freshly chopped coriander makes a good garnish for this dish.

CHINESE PAK CHOI & PRAWNS

345 calories per serving

Ingredients

- 125g/4oz wholemeal microwavable rice
- 1 pak choi
- 60ml/¼ cup chicken stock
- 1 tsp olive oil
- 1 garlic clove, crushed
- ½ onion, sliced
- 1 tsp freshly grated ginger
- 150g/5oz shelled raw king prawns
- 1 tsp soy sauce
- ½ tsp Chinese five spice powder
- Pinch crushed chilli flakes
- Salt & pepper to taste

Method

1 Shred the pak choi and gently wilt in a frying pan with the chicken stock for a few minutes until tender.

2 Heat the olive oil in a frying pan and sauté the garlic, onions & ginger for a minute or two.

3 Add the prawns, soy sauce, Chinese five spice powder & chilli flakes and cook until the prawns are pink.

4 Check the prawns are cooked through. Add the rice to the pan and heat through for a couple of minutes.

5 Quickly toss through the pak choi. Season and serve immediately.

CHEFS NOTE
Pak choi is a readily available oriental cabbage but any type of cabbage will work well.

PEPPERS & STEAK

385
calories per serving

Ingredients

- 150g/5oz sirloin steak
- 2 tsp olive oil
- ½ tsp paprika
- ½ onion, sliced
- 1 garlic clove, crushed

- 1 red or yellow pepper, deseeded & sliced
- 125g/4oz cherry tomatoes
- 1 baby gem lettuces, shredded
- 25g/1oz feta cheese, crumbled
- Salt & pepper to taste

Method

1 Trim any fat off the steak. Lightly brush with a little of the olive oil & all the paprika. Season and put a frying pan on a high heat.

2 In another pan gently sauté the peppers, onions & garlic in the rest of the olive oil for 5-7 minutes or until tender.

3 Place the steak in the smoking hot dry pan and cook for 1-2 minutes each side, or to your liking. Leave to rest for 3 minutes and then finely slice.

4 Halve the tomatoes & shred the lettuces. Add the peppers, crumble the feta cheese and combine on plates.

5 Place the sliced steak on top. Season and serve.

CHEFS NOTE

You could choose to use Stilton cheese instead of feta for this lovely fresh recipe.

MEXICAN BEAN SOUP

280
calories per serving

Ingredients

- 2 tsp olive oil
- ½ garlic clove, crushed
- ¼ onion, sliced
- 120ml/½ cup vegetable stock
- 120ml/½ cup tomato passata/sieved tomatoes
- 50g/2oz vine ripened tomatoes, chopped
- 100g/3½oz tinned black-eyed beans, drained
- 2 tsp lime juice
- 1 tbsp freshly chopped coriander/cilantro
- Salt & pepper to taste

Method

1 Gently sauté the onion and garlic in the olive oil for a few minutes.

2 Add all the ingredients, except the chopped coriander, to the pan. Bring to the boil, cover and leave to simmer for 10 minutes or until everything is tender.

3 Blend to your preferred consistency, season and serve with coriander sprinkled over the top.

CHEFS NOTE
Use whichever beans you prefer for this filling soup.

MED SALAD SOUP

289 calories per serving

Ingredients

- 2 tsp olive oil
- 2 shallots, sliced
- 75g/3oz courgettes/zucchini, chopped
- 125g/4oz peas
- 50g/2oz spinach
- 1 celery stalk, chopped
- ¼ fennel bulb chopped
- 1 baby gem lettuce, shredded
- 250ml/1 cup vegetable stock
- 120ml/½ cup milk
- Salt & pepper to taste

Method

1 Heat a pan and gently sauté the shallots and courgettes in the olive oil for a few minutes.

2 Add all the other ingredients, except the shredded lettuce and milk, to the pan. Bring to the boil, cover and leave to gently simmer for 8-10 minutes or until everything is tender.

3 Blend to your preferred consistency stir through the milk and add the shredded lettuce. Stir through, season and serve immediately.

CHEFS NOTE
Adding fresh lettuce after cooking gives a lovely crunch to this unusual Mediterranean soup. You could add some finely chopped radishes too.

SEAFOOD COCKTAIL SALAD

389 calories per serving

Ingredients

- 1 tbsp mayonnaise
- 1 dash Tabasco sauce
- ½ tsp lemon juice
- 1 tsp freshly chopped chives
- 100g/3½oz cooked & peeled prawns
- 100g/3½oz cooked crabmeat
- 1 baby gem lettuce, shredded
- ½ ripe avocado, peeled, stoned & diced
- ¼ cucumber, diced
- Salt & pepper to taste

Method

1 Mix together the mayonnaise, Tabasco sauce, lemon juice, chives, prawns and crabmeat until everything is really well combined.

2 In a separate bowl gently combine the shredded lettuce, avocado & cucumber to make a salad.

3 Pile the dressed prawns and crabmeat on top and serve.

CHEFS NOTE
Sprinkle with a little paprika and serve with lemon wedges.

TUNA BEAN SALAD

450 calories per serving

Ingredients

- ½ cucumber, finely sliced into matchsticks
- ½ tsp honey
- 2 tsp rice wine vinegar
- Pinch dried chilli flakes
- ½ red onion, finely chopped
- 75g/3oz cherry tomatoes, halved
- 200g/7oz tinned borlotti beans, drained & rinsed
- 125g/5oz tinned tuna, drained
- ¼ avocado, cubed
- 25g/5oz rocket
- Salt & pepper to taste

Method

1 Place the cucumber in a frying pan and gently warm over a low heat. Add the rice wine vinegar, honey & chilli flakes. Simmer for a few minutes and set aside to cool.

2 Meanwhile mix together the red onion, beans, tomatoes & tuna in a large bowl. Add the cooled cucumber, toss with the avocado and rocket and serve.

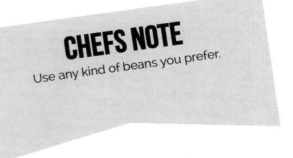

CHEFS NOTE
Use any kind of beans you prefer.

NUTTY SPROUT SALAD

215 calories per serving

Ingredients

- 150g/5oz prepared Brussels sprouts
- 2 tsp butter
- 3 shallots, sliced
- 1 tbsp slivered almonds
- A drizzle of extra virgin olive oil
- Salt & pepper to taste

Method

1 Slice the sprouts really thinly so they fall into shreds.

2 Heat the butter in a frying pan and gently sauté the shallots and almonds for a few minutes until the shallots are soft and golden.

3 Meanwhile plunge the shredded sprouts into salted boiling water for 2 minutes. Drain and rinse through with cold water. Add to the onion pan and toss until piping hot and cooked through.

4 Season with plenty of salt & freshly ground pepper and a drizzle of olive oil.

CHEFS NOTE
It is thought almonds can reduce the rise in blood sugar and insulin levels after meals.

NAPOLITANO SPAGHETTI

330 calories per serving

Ingredients

- 75g/13z wholemeal spaghetti
- 2 tsp olive oil
- 125g/4oz cherry tomatoes, roughly chopped
- 50g/2oz pitted black olives, roughly chopped
- 1 stalk of celery, finely chopped

- ½ onion, finely chopped
- 1 garlic clove, crushed
- 1 tbsp tomato puree
- 1 tbsp freshly chopped basil
- Salt & pepper to taste

Method

1 Heat the oil and gently sauté the tomatoes, olives, celery, onions, garlic, tomato puree & basil for 10 minutes or until the tomatoes lose their shape and combine to make a sauce.

2 Whilst the sauce is cooking place the spaghetti in a pan of salted boiling water until tender. Drain the cooked pasta and add to the frying pan.

3 Toss well, season & serve.

CHEFS NOTE
You could cook the sauce for longer if you have the time to increase the richness of the dish.

FLAKED SALMON FILLET & SAVOY CABBAGE

275 calories per serving

Ingredients

- 150g/5oz skinless salmon fillet
- ¼ savoy cabbage, shredded
- 1 tsp olive oil
- 1 garlic clove, crushed
- 2 tsp freshly chopped chives

- 2 tsp low fat crème fraiche
- 2 tsp horseradish sauce
- 1 tsp lemon juice
- Salt & pepper to taste

Method

1 Season the salmon fillet and place under a preheated grill for 10-12 minutes or until cooked through. Flake and put to one side to cool.

2 Meanwhile steam the cabbage for 8-10 minutes or until the cabbage is tender. Heat the oil and garlic in a saucepan and gently sauté for a minute or two. Add the cooked cabbage, stir well and cook for a minute or two longer.

3 Gently combine together the chives, crème fraiche, horseradish sauce, lemon juice & flaked salmon.

4 Divide the dressed salmon and sautéed cabbage onto a plate, season & serve.

CHEFS NOTE
Feel free to use precooked salmon fillets if you are short of time.

DOLCELATTE CHICKEN SALAD

370 calories per serving

Ingredients

- 150g/5oz cooked chicken breast, sliced
- 75g/3oz cherry tomatoes
- 25g/1oz Dolcelatte cheese
- ½ ripe avocado peeled, stoned & cubed
- 1 tsp extra virgin olive oil

- 1 tsp cider vinegar
- 1 tsp low fat crème fraiche
- ½ tsp paprika
- 300g/11oz watercress
- Salt & pepper to taste

Method

1 Halve the cherry tomatoes and crumble the Dolcelatte cheese.

2 Combine together the olive oil, vinegar, crème fraiche & paprika to make a dressing.

3 Toss the dressing, tomatoes, cheese, avocado & watercress together in a large bowl.

4 Arrange the chicken slices on top. Season and serve.

CHEFS NOTE
Feta cheese also works well in this recipe.

THE *Skinny*
15 MINUTE MEALS
& *HIIT* WORKOUT PLAN

DINNER

FRESH CHICKEN KEBABS

420 calories per serving

Ingredients

- ½ garlic clove, crushed
- 1 tbsp olive oil
- 2 tsp lime juice
- 150g/5oz skinless chicken breast, cubed
- 1 red pepper, deseeded & cut onto chunks
- 1 red onion, peeled and cut into chunks
- 8 button mushrooms
- 2 tbsp freshly chopped coriander/cilantro
- Salt & pepper to taste
- Metal skewers

Method

1 Preheat the grill to a medium/high heat.

2 Mix together the garlic, olive oil & lime juice in a bowl. Season the chicken and vegetables and add to the oil. Combine well and skewer each piece in turn to make 2 chicken and vegetable kebabs.

3 Place under the grill and cook for 5-6 minutes each side or until the chicken is cooked through and piping hot. Remove from the grill, season and serve with chopped coriander sprinkled over the top.

CHEFS NOTE

Substitute the coriander with any fresh herbs you prefer.

LAMB KOFTA

410 calories per serving

Ingredients

- 125g/4oz lean lamb mince
- ½ tsp each ground cumin & coriander
- 1 garlic clove, crushed
- 1 tsp olive oil
- 1 cereal pitta bread
- 1 baby gem lettuce, shredded
- 1 tbsp fat free Greek yoghurt
- 1 tsp mint sauce
- 2 kebab skewers
- Salt & pepper to taste

Method

1 Preheat the grill.

2 Place the lamb mince, cumin, coriander, garlic & salt in a food processor and pulse to combine. Scoop out the mixture and use your hands to form into 2 balls.

3 Roll the balls into oval shapes and thread lengthways onto the skewers. Spray with a brush with olive oil, place under a preheated medium grill and cook for 8-12 minutes or until cooked through.

4 Mix the yoghurt and mint sauce together.

5 Warm the pitta bread under the grill, take the koftas off the skewers and place in the pittas along with the shredded lettuce & mint yoghurt.

CHEFS NOTE

Cereal pitta bread is made using a combination cereals including Linseed, Sunflower Seeds, Chunky Oats, Quinoa and Rye.

SOYA BEAN & TOFU PENNE

425 calories per serving

Ingredients

- 50g/2oz tofu
- 75g/3oz buckwheat penne
- 1 tsp olive oil
- 1 garlic cloves, crushed
- 50g/2oz soya beans
- 50g/2oz fresh peas
- 1 tbsp low fat crème fraiche
- 1 tsp freshly chopped mint
- Salt & pepper to taste

Method

1 First cube the tofu and dry off as much as possible.

2 Begin cooking the penne in a pan of boiling water until tender.

3 Meanwhile heat the olive oil in a high-sided frying pan and stir-fry the tofu for a few minutes on a high heat.

4 Reduce the heat, add the garlic, soya beans and peas and sauté for a few minutes. When the peas and beans are cooked through stir in the crème fraiche and mint.

5 Drain the cooked penne and add to the pan.

6 Toss well, season & serve with lots of freshly ground black pepper.

CHEFS NOTE

The dryer the tofu is, the better it will stir-fry.

PESTO & BUCKWHEAT SPAGHETTI

420 calories per serving

Ingredients

- 75g/3oz buckwheat noodles/spaghetti
- 2 shallots, sliced
- 1 tbsp pesto

- 75g/3oz watercress
- 1 tsp Parmesan shavings
- Salt & pepper to taste

Method

1 Cook the buckwheat pasta in a pan of boiling water until tender.

2 Meanwhile heat the oil and gently sauté the shallots in a high-sided frying pan whilst the pasta cooks.

3 Drain the cooked pasta and add to the frying pan along with the parsley pesto. Toss well.

4 Sit the past on a bed of watercress, sprinkle Parmesan, season & serve.

CHEFS NOTE
Shop bought pesto is fine for this simple supper.

SOYA BEAN & PRAWN NOODLES

480 calories per serving

Ingredients

- 1 tsp olive oil
- ½ red chilli, deseeded & finely chopped
- 1 garlic clove, crushed garlic
- 1 tsp grated fresh ginger
- 125g/4oz shelled king prawns
- 1 red pepper

- 2 tbsp soy sauce
- 75g/5oz soya beans
- 75g/3oz buckwheat noodles
- 1 bunch spring onions/scallions
- Salt & pepper to taste

Method

1 Heat the olive oil in a frying pan or wok and gently sauté the chilli, garlic and ginger for a minute or two. Add the prawns and cook for a few minutes until they begin to pink up.

2 Meanwhile quickly de-seed & slice the red pepper. Add to the pan along with the soya beans and soy sauce.

3 Stir-fry for 3-4 minutes whilst you cook the noodles in boiling water until tender.

4 Check the prawns are cooked through and when the noodles are ready, add to the pan. Combine for a minute or two.

5 Slice the spring onions and use these as a fresh garnish.

CHEFS NOTE
Buckwheat is rich in Rutin which has anti-inflammatory properties.

SESAME VEGGIE NOODLES

310 calories per serving

Ingredients

- 2 tsp fish sauce
- 1 tsp sesame oil
- 1 tbsp soy sauce
- 1 tsp lime juice
- 1 tsp honey
- ½ tsp sesame seeds
- ½ red chilli, deseeded & finely chopped
- 1 tbsp freshly chopped coriander
- 150g/5oz wholewheat straight-to-wok egg noodles
- Salt & pepper to taste

Method

1 Mix together the fish sauce, sesame oil, soy sauce, lime juice, honey, sesame seeds & chillies to make a dressing.

2 Gently warm the dressing in a saucepan and add the noodles. Cook for a few minutes until the noodles are piping hot. Sprinkle with chopped coriander, season & serve.

CHEFS NOTE
Chopped fresh basil makes a good addition to this dish too.

CHICKEN CHOW MEIN

470 calories per serving

Ingredients

- 100g/3½oz skinless chicken breast, sliced
- ½ tsp Chinese 5 spice powder
- 1 tsp olive oil
- 1 garlic clove, crushed
- 1 carrots, cut into match sticks
- ½ onion, sliced
- ¼ pointed cabbage, shredded
- 2 tsp rice wine vinegar
- 2 tsp fish sauce
- 1 tbsp sweet chilli sauce
- 2 tbp soy sauce
- 150g/5oz beansprouts
- 150g/5oz wholewheat straight-to-wok egg noodles
- Salt & pepper to taste

Method

1 Mix the chicken breast and 5 spice powder together.

2 Heat the olive oil in a deep sided frying pan and gently sauté the garlic, carrots and onions for a few minutes until softened.

3 Add the chicken and cabbage to the pan and cook for 5-7 minutes or until the chicken is cooked through.

4 Mix together the rice wine vinegar, fish sauce, sweet chilli sauce and soy sauce together to make a combined sauce. Add the beansprouts, noodles & sauce to the pan and cook until the dish is piping hot. Season & serve.

CHEFS NOTE
Chopped spring onions make a perfect garnish for this dish.

PORK, PINEAPPLE & PEPPERS

450
calories per
serving

Ingredients

- 1 tsp olive oil
- 1 yellow pepper, deseeded & sliced
- ½ onion, sliced
- ½ red chilli, deseeded & finely chopped
- 125g/5oz pork tenderloin, diced
- 2 tbsp pineapple juice
- 50g/2oz pineapple chunks, drained and chopped
- 1 tbsp soy sauce
- 1 tsp lime juice
- 150g/ 5oz wholewheat straight-to-wok egg noodles
- 1 tbsp freshly chopped flat leaf parsley
- Salt & pepper to taste

Method

1 Heat the olive oil in a frying pan or wok and gently sauté the peppers, onions and chopped chilli for a few minutes until softened.

2 Add the pork, pineapple juice, pineapple chunks, soy sauce & lime juice and continue to stir-fry until the pork is cooked through.

3 Add the noodles to the pan and cook until piping hot. Sprinkle with chopped parsley & serve.

CHEFS NOTE
Prawns are a good alternative to pork in this recipe.

HOISIN & CASHEW CHICKEN STIR-FRY

470 calories per serving

Ingredients

- 125g/4oz wholemeal microwavable rice
- 125g/4oz skinless chicken breast, chopped
- 1 tsp honey
- 1 tsp olive oil
- ½ onion, chopped
- 1 red pepper, deseeded & sliced
- 50g/2oz mangetout, trimmed
- 50g/2oz baby sweetcorn, chopped
- 1 pak choi, shredded
- 50g/2oz cashew nuts, halved
- 1 tbsp soy sauce
- ½ tsp cornflour
- 1 tbsp hoisin sauce
- Salt & pepper to taste

Method

1 Mix the chicken and honey together.

2 Heat the olive oil in a frying pan or wok and gently sauté the chopped onions, peppers, mangetout & sweetcorn for a few minutes until softened.

3 Add the chicken, pak choi & nuts to the pan and cook for 4-5 minutes or until the chicken is cooked through.

4 Mix together the soy sauce, cornflour and hoisin sauce to make a smooth paste (add a little water if needed). Add to the pan, turn up the heat and cook until the dish is piping hot and the chicken is cooked through.

5 Add the rice to the pan, warm through. Combine well, season and serve immediately.

CHEFS NOTE

Feel free to substitute other vegetables in place of mangetout and baby corn.

CHICKEN & NOODLE BROTH

480 calories per serving

Ingredients

- 50g/2oz peas
- 1 garlic clove, crushed
- 250ml/1 cup chicken stock
- 1 tsp freshly grated ginger
- 1 tbsp soy sauce
- 50g/2oz spinach, chopped

- 150g/5oz wholewheat straight-to-wok egg noodles
- 100g/3½oz cooked chicken breast, shredded
- 1 tsp coconut cream
- 2 spring onions, chopped
- Salt & pepper to taste

Method

1 Place all the ingredients, except the chicken, coconut cream and spring onions, in a saucepan.

2 Gently cook for a 5-7 minutes. Add the shredded chicken and coconut cream, combine well and keep on the heat until the chicken is piping hot.

3 Season and serve with the chopped spring onions sprinkled over the top.

CHEFS NOTE
Using cooked chicken means you can shred the meat finely before adding to the pan, which benefits the texture of the broth.

PRAWN & PARSLEY QUINOA

295 calories per serving

Ingredients

- 50g/2oz quinoa
- 1 tsp olive oil
- 1 garlic clove, crushed
- 200g/7oz raw, shelled king prawns
- 1 tbsp lemon juice
- 2 tbsp freshly chopped flat leaf parsley
- 1 romaine lettuce shredded
- Salt & pepper to taste

Method

1 Put the quinoa in a saucepan, cover and cook in boiling water for about 10 minutes or until it is tender. (Cook in vegetable stock if you wish rather than water.)

2 Meanwhile heat the olive oil and gently sauté the garlic, prawns & lemon juice whilst the quinoa cooks.

3 When the prawns are cooked through and the quinoa is tender, drain any excess liquid from the quinoa and add to the frying pan with the prawns.

4 Toss well. Arrange the shredded lettuce in a shallow bowl and pile the prawns and quinoa on top. Sprinkle with chopped parsley and serve.

CHEFS NOTE

Prawns, lemon and garlic are a match made in heaven. Add more garlic if you prefer a stronger taste.

SUNDRIED TOMATO & CAPER GRAINS

260 calories per serving

Ingredients

- 75g/3oz quinoa
- 200g/7oz ripe cherry tomatoes
- 1 tbsp capers
- 1 tbsp sultanas
- 2 tsp olive oil

- ½ garlic clove, crushed
- 3 sundried tomatoes (from a jar)
- 1 tbsp freshly chopped basil
- Salt & pepper to taste

Method

1 Put the quinoa in a saucepan, cover and cook in boiling water for about 10 minutes or until it's tender. (Cook in vegetable stock if you wish rather than water.)

2 Half the cherry tomatoes and roughly chop the capers, sultanas and sundried tomatoes.

3 Heat the olive oil and gently sauté the garlic, cherry tomatoes, capers, sultanas and sundried tomatoes whilst the quinoa cooks. When the quinoa grains are tender drain any excess water and add to the frying pan.

4 Toss well and serve with chopped basil on top.

CHEFS NOTE
This is good served on a bed of rocket and spinach.

ZUCCHINI & BLACK OLIVE BULGUR WHEAT

345 calories per serving

Ingredients

- 75g/3oz bulgur wheat
- 100g/3½oz baby courgettes/zucchini
- 8 pitted black olives, sliced
- ½ onion, chopped
- 1 garlic clove, crushed
- 1 tbsp lemon juice
- 2 tsp olive oil
- Lemon wedges to serve
- 1 tbsp freshly chopped mint
- Salt & pepper to taste

Method

1 Cook the bulgur wheat in boiling water for 10 minutes or until tender. (Cook in vegetable stock if you wish rather than water.)

2 Use a vegetable peeler to cut the courgettes into ribbons. Gently sauté the sliced olives, chopped onions, garlic, lemon juice and courgette ribbons in the olive oil for a few minutes.

3 When the bulgur wheat is ready drain off any excess water. Fluff the bulgur wheat with a fork and pile into the onion and courgette pan. Mix well and serve on a plate with fresh lemon wedges on the side and chopped mint sprinkled over the top.

CHEFS NOTE
You could use chopped basil or coriander in place of mint if you like.

FRESH MINT FISH

340 calories per serving

Ingredients

- 150g/5oz skinless, boneless fish fillet
- ½ garlic clove, crushed
- 2 tsp extra virgin olive oil
- 2 tsp lemon juice
- 1 tbsp freshly chopped mint
- 2 large ripe beef tomatoes, thickly sliced
- ½ red onion finely sliced into rounds
- 50g/2oz mozzarella cheese, sliced
- Salt & pepper to taste

Method

1 Preheat the grill to a medium/high heat.

2 Mix together the garlic, olive oil & lemon juice and brush on either side of the fish fillet. Place the fish under the grill and cook for 2-3 minutes each side or until the fillet is cooked through.

3 Meanwhile arrange the sliced tomatoes, red onion and mozzarella on the plate. Sit the cooked fish to the side and sprinkle the mint all over.

CHEFS NOTE
Use whichever fish you prefer. Oily is best.

PRAWN & PINEAPPLE SKEWERS

320 calories per serving

Ingredients

- ½ garlic clove, crushed
- 1 tbsp extra virgin olive oil
- 2 tsp lime juice
- 150g/5oz large king prawns
- 75g/3oz pineapple chunks
- 1 red pepper, cut into chunks
- Salt & pepper to taste
- Metal skewers

Method

1 Preheat the grill to a medium/high heat.

2 Mix together the garlic, olive oil & lime juice in a bowl. Season the prawns, peppers and pineapple pieces and add to the bowl. Combine well and skewer each piece in turn to make two large kebabs. Place under the grill and cook for 4-5 minutes each side or until the prawns are pink and cooked through.

3 Remove from the grill, season and serve.

CHEFS NOTE
These skewers are great served with wild rice and a dollop of Greek yoghurt.

CHICKEN, RAISINS & RICE

415 calories per serving

Ingredients

- 125g/4oz wholemeal microwavable rice
- 1 tbsp olive oil
- 1 garlic clove, crushed
- ½ onion, chopped
- 50g/2oz raisins

- 125g/4oz skinless chicken breast, diced
- 1 beef tomatoes, toughly chopped
- 1 tbsp freshly chopped coriander
- Salt & pepper to taste

Method

1 Heat the oil in a frying pan and gently sauté the onions & garlic for a few minutes until softened.

2 Add the raisins, chicken & chopped tomatoes and cook for a few minutes until the chicken is cooked through.

3 Add the rice to the pan, combine and heat through for a couple of minutes. Remove from the heat, stir well and serve with chopped coriander sprinkled over the top.

CHEFS NOTE
Feel free to toss the coriander through the dish rather than serving as a garnish if you prefer.

SPINACH, PRAWNS & PINE NUTS

380 calories per serving

Ingredients

- 125g/4oz wholemeal microwavable rice
- 1 tsp olive oil
- ½ onion, chopped
- 1 tsp freshly grated ginger
- ½ green chilli, deseeded & finely sliced
- 1 garlic clove, crushed
- 2 tsp lime juice
- 125g/4oz raw, peeled king prawns
- 100g/3½oz spinach
- 60ml/¼ cup chicken stock
- 1 tbsp pine nuts
- Salt & pepper to taste

Method

1 Heat the olive oil in a frying pan and gently sauté the onions, garlic, sliced chilli & ginger for a few minutes until softened.

2 Add the lime juice, prawns, spinach & stock and cook for 5-8 minutes on a high heat until the stock has reduced and the prawns are cooked through.

3 Tip the rice into the pan along with pine nuts and cook for a minute or two.

4 Remove from the heat, stir well, season & serve.

CHEFS NOTE
If you have time, gently toast the pine nuts in a dry pan for a couple of minutes until golden brown.

LAMB KHEEMA GHOTALA

480 calories per serving

Ingredients

- 125g/4oz wholemeal microwavable rice
- 2 tsp olive oil
- ½ onion, sliced
- 1 garlic clove, crushed
- 1 large beef tomatoes, roughly chopped
- 2 tsp curry powder
- 125g/4oz lean lamb mince
- 1 free range egg
- Salt & pepper to taste

Method

1 Heat the oil in a frying pan and gently sauté the onions & garlic for a few minutes until softened.

2 Add the tomatoes, curry powder and mince to the pan. Increase the heat and brown for 2-3 minutes.

3 Reduce the heat, stir well and cook for 6-8 minutes or until the mince is cooked through. Add the rice and heat through.

4 Lightly beat the egg with a fork and add to the lamb mince. Stir though to scramble for a minute or two.

5 Season and serve.

CHEFS NOTE

For something completely different you could leave out the rice and serve this dish as a spicy Indian breakfast!

STEAK & DRESSED GREENS

450
calories per
serving

Ingredients

- 125g/4oz mini salad potatoes, quartered
- 1 sirloin steak weighing 125g/4oz
- 100g/3½oz spring greens
- 1 tsp olive oil
- 1 tsp runny honey
- 1 orange, zest & juice
- Salt & pepper to taste

Method

1 Place the potatoes and spring greens into a saucepan of salted water and cook for 6-8 minutes or until tender.

2 Trim any fat off the steak, season and lightly brush with olive oil.

3 Place the steak in a smoking-hot pan and cook for 1-2 minutes each side, or to your liking.

4 When the steak is cooked, put to one side to rest for 3 minutes.

5 Combine together the olive oil, honey, orange juice & zest to make a dressing.

6 Drain the potatoes and greens and place in a bowl with the dressing. Season and combine well.

7 Serve the steak with the dressed potatoes & greens on the side.

CHEFS NOTE

You could add some fresh oregano to serve with the steaks if you like.

CHICKEN & WILTED LETTUCE IN OYSTER SAUCE

420 calories per serving

Ingredients

- 125g/4oz wholemeal microwavable rice
- 1 tsp olive oil
- 1 red pepper, deseeded & sliced
- 75g/3oz mushrooms, sliced
- 125g/4oz skinless chicken breast, chopped
- 1 tbsp oyster sauce
- ½ iceberg lettuce, shredded
- Salt & pepper to taste

Method

1 Heat the olive oil in a frying pan or wok and gently sauté the peppers and mushrooms for a few minutes until softened.

2 Add the chicken and oyster sauce to the pan and fry on a high heat for 4-5 minutes or until the chicken is cooked through. Add the rice to the pan and cook through.

3 At the end of this cooking time plunge the shredded lettuce into salted boiling water for 10 seconds.

4 Season and serve immediately on top of the blanched lettuce.

CHEFS NOTE
Blanching the lettuce for just 10 seconds will slightly wilt the salad leaves.

SPICED CHICKEN & LO-CARB RICE

480 calories per serving

Ingredients

- 50g/2oz red onion, chopped
- 75g/3oz green beans
- 1 garlic clove, crushed
- 1 tbsp extra virgin olive oil
- 125g/4oz cherry tomatoes, chopped
- 1 tbsp sultanas
- 150g/5oz chicken breast, sliced
- 2 tsp medium curry powder
- 1 tbsp coconut cream
- 2 tbsp flat leaf parsley, chopped
- 200g/7oz cauliflower florets
- 1 tbsp chopped coriander/cilantro
- Salt & pepper to taste

Method

1 Get the onions, green beans, garlic, cherry tomatoes & sultanas gently cooking in a frying pan with the olive oil. Sauté for a few minutes and then add the chicken & curry powder (add a little more olive oil if needed).

2 Cook for a few minutes until the chicken is cooked thorough then stir through the coconut cream and parsley.

3 Meanwhile place the cauliflower florets in a food processor and pulse a few times until the cauliflower is the size of rice grains.

4 Place the 'rice' in a microwavable dish, cover and cook on full power for about 90 seconds minutes or until it's piping hot.

5 Tip the 'rice' into a shallow bowl. Serve the chicken and vegetables over the top sprinkled with chopped coriander.

CHEFS NOTE
Prawns or pork are also good in this simple spiced dish.

POMEGRANATE HERBED QUINOA

455 calories per serving

Ingredients

- 75g/3oz quinoa
- 3 tbsp pomegranate seeds
- 2 tsp lemon juice
- 1 tbsp extra virgin olive oil
- 1 tbsp fresh mint, chopped
- 2 tbsp flat leaf parsley, chopped
- 50g/2oz carrot, grated
- 50g/2oz celery, sliced
- 50g/2oz feta cheese, crumbled
- 1 tbsp balsamic vinegar
- Salt & pepper to taste

Method

1 Put the quinoa in a saucepan, cover and cook in boiling water for about 10 minutes or until it's tender. (Cook in vegetable stock if you wish, rather than water.)

2 Once the quinoa is ready, drain it and fluff with a fork. Combine with the pomegranate seeds, lemon juice, olive oil, mint and parsley.

3 Pile the grated carrot and sliced celery on top. Add the crumbled feta cheese and drizzle the balsamic vinegar over the cheese.

4 Season and serve.

CHEFS NOTE
Add as much balsamic vinegar as you like to this crunchy quinoa salad.

VIETNAMESE PRAWNS

485 calories per serving

Ingredients

- 125g/4oz wholemeal microwavable rice
- 2 tsp extra virgin olive oil
- 50g/2oz red onion
- 50g/2oz green beans, chopped
- 2 garlic cloves, crushed
- 1 red chilli, sliced (leave the seeds in)
- 2 tbsp lime juice

- 2 tbsp fish sauce
- ½ tsp brown sugar
- 125g/4oz cooked prawns, chopped
- 1 tbsp flat leaf parsley, chopped
- 50g/2oz spinach
- Salt & pepper to taste

Method

1 Heat up a frying pan with the olive oil and start sautéing the onions for a few minutes until softened

2 While the onions are cooking combine the garlic cloves, chilli, lime juice, fish sauce and brown sugar to make a spicy, sweet & sour dressing.

3 Tip the rice and prawns into the pan with the onions and warm for a few minutes until everything is piping hot. Add the spinach for the last 60 seconds until it is gently wilted.

4 Tip the prawns & rice into a shallow bowl, drizzle the dressing over the top and sprinkle with parsley.

CHEFS NOTE
Balance the chilli, lime and sugar to suit your own taste in the fiery Vietnamese dressing.

EDAMAME CHICKEN

410 calories per serving

Ingredients

- 2 tsp olive oil
- ½ red onion, sliced
- ½ garlic clove, crushed
- 1 celery stalk, chopped
- 150g/5oz skinless chicken breast, thickly sliced
- 1 tbsp fresh chopped marjoram
- 60ml/¼ cup chicken stock/broth
- 75g/3oz fresh edamame beans
- 125g/4oz spinach leaves
- Salt & pepper to taste

Method

1 In a saucepan gently sauté the onion, celery and garlic in the olive oil for a few minutes until softened.

2 Add the chicken, marjoram & stock and leave to gently simmer for 8-10 minutes or until the chicken is cooked through and the stock has reduced.

3 Add the edamame and cook for a minute or two.

4 Add the spinach and stir for a minute or two until wilted.

5 Season and serve.

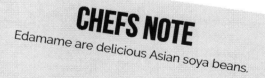

CHEFS NOTE
Edamame are delicious Asian soya beans.

FENNEL, CHICKEN & BEANS

485 calories per serving

Ingredients

- 2 tsp olive oil
- ¼ onion, sliced
- ½ fennel bulb, finely sliced
- 1 garlic cloves, crushed
- 200g/7oz tinned flageolet beans, drained
- 60ml/¼ cup chicken stock/broth
- 1 tbsp freshly chopped basil
- 150g/5oz skinless chicken breast, thickly sliced
- 1 tsp Parmesan shavings
- Salt & pepper to taste

Method

1 Gently sauté the onion, fennel and garlic in the olive oil for a few minutes until softened. Add the beans, chicken & stock and leave to gently simmer for 10 minutes or until the chicken is cooked through and the stock has reduced.

2 Sprinkle with chopped basil and Parmesan shaving. Season and serve.

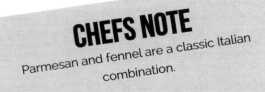

CHEFS NOTE
Parmesan and fennel are a classic Italian combination.

HiiT Plan WORKOUTS

High Intensity Interval Training is a super fast and really effective way to workout. The short but intense bursts of exercise with rest in between makes your heart work harder and so increases cardio strength, improves metabolism and as a result helps your body burn more calories both during and after your workout. HiiT can also help control blood sugar levels.

It's a very efficient way to train to build a leaner, fitter body and because no equipment is required you can workout at home or just about anywhere.

We have compiled **4** core workouts to perform throughout each week. Choose one workout to perform per day and use the remaining 3 days to rest. Try to alternate between training and rest days. Each workout lasts for approximately 15 mins and a simple explanation of how to correctly perform each exercise in the set is explained in the following pages.

It's very important to warm up your muscles and joints before beginning any exercise to prevent injury and to make sure you perform each repetition to the best of your ability. Stretch for at least 2 minutes before your workout (see page 94 for stretches), then warm up by jogging on the spot for two minutes.

Always cool down and stretch again at the end of your workout.

Tips

- Warm up and cool down before and after each workout
- Have a bottle of water to drink from between sets
- Remember to breathe through each exercise
- Keep your core tight & give maximum effort
- Focus on maintaining correct posture & form for each exercise

HiiT WORKOUT ONE

- Exercise 1: **HIGH KNEES** 20 secs | 10 secs rest
- Exercise 2: **BODYWEIGHT SQUATS** 20 secs | 10 secs rest
- Exercise 3: **JUMPING JACKS** 20 secs | 10 secs rest
- Exercise 4: **SIDE LUNGE** 20 secs | 10 secs rest
- Exercise 5: **TRICEP DIPS** 20 secs | 10 secs rest
- Exercise 6: **MOUNTAIN CLIMBERS** 20 secs | 10 sec rest
- Exercise 7: **BUTT KICKS** 20 secs | 2 minute rest

Repeat for 2 more sets

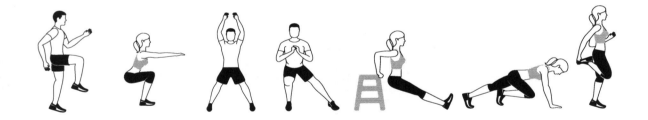

Perform each exercise as many times as possible within 20 seconds. Rest for 10 seconds then perform the next exercise again for 20 secs with a 10 sec rest in between exercises. Repeat until all 7 exercises have been completed.

Rest for 2 minutes then repeat the whole set two more times with a 2 minute rest in between.

Remember that these are high intensity workouts so try to push yourself to get as many repetitions of each exercise with the correct form within the 20 second period.

High KNEES

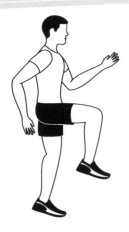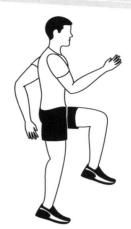

Stand straight with the feet hip width apart, looking straight ahead and arms hanging down by your side. Jump from one foot to the other at the same time lifting your knees as high as possible, hip height is advisable. The arms should be following the motion. Try holding your hands just above the hips so that your knees touch the palms of your hands as you lift your knees.

Bodyweight SQUATS

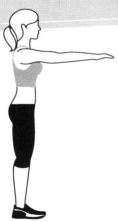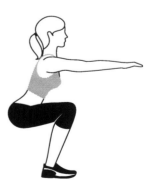

Stand with your feet shoulder width apart with your arms extended in front of you. Begin the movement by flexing your knees and hips, sitting back with your hips until your thighs are parallel with the floor in the full squat position. Quickly reverse the motion until you return to the starting position. As you keep your head and chest up.

Jumping JACKS

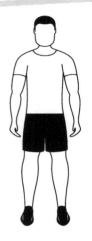 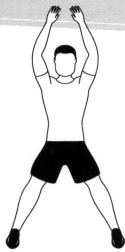

Stand with your feet together and your hands down by your side. In one motion jump your feet out to the side and raise your arms above your head. Immediately reverse by jumping back to the starting position.

Side LUNGE

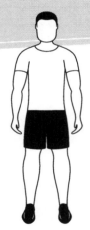 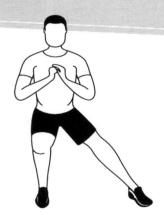

Stand with your knees and hips slightly bent, feet shoulder-width apart and the head and chest up. Keeping your left leg straight, step out to the side with your right leg and bend at your right knee transferring weight to your right side. Extend through the right leg to return to the starting position. Repeat on the left leg.

Tricep DIPS

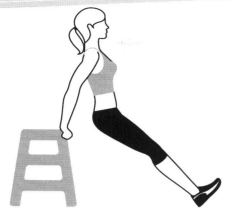 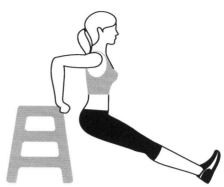

Position your hands shoulder-width apart on a secure bench or stable chair. Slide off the front of the bench with your legs extended out in front of you. Straighten your arms, keeping a slight bend in your elbows. Slowly bend your elbows to lower your body toward the floor until your elbows are at about a 90-degree angle. At this point press down into the bench or chair to straighten your elbows, returning to the starting position.

Mountain CLIMBER

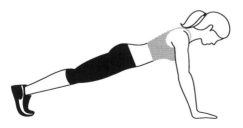 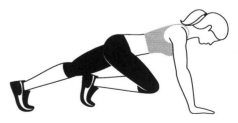

Begin in a pushup position, with your weight supported by your hands and toes. Flexing the knee and hip, bring one leg towards the corresponding arm. Explosively reverse the positions of your legs, extending the bent leg until the leg is straight and supported by the toe, and bringing the other foot up with the hip and knee flexed. Repeat in an alternating fashion.

Butt KICKS

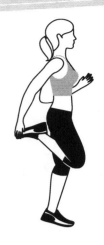 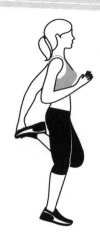

Stand with your legs shoulder-width apart and your arms bent. Flex the right knee and kick your right heel up toward your glutes. Bring the right foot back down while flexing your left knee and kicking your left foot up toward your glutes. Repeat in a continuous movement.

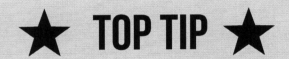

★ **TOP TIP** ★

Warm up properly. By warming up your muscles you will reduce the chances of injury or strain. Warm up with jogging on the spot, gentle jumping jacks and stretches (see page 94) for at least 2 minutes.

- Exercise 1: **BURPEES** 20 secs | 10 secs rest
- Exercise 2: **JAB SQUATS** 20 secs | 10 secs rest
- Exercise 3: **MUMMY KICKS** 20 secs | 10 secs rest
- Exercise 4: **SIDE SKATER** 20 secs | 10 secs rest
- Exercise 5: **TUCK JUMP** 20 secs | 10 secs rest
- Exercise 6: **SPRINTS** 20 secs | 10 sec rest
- Exercise 7: **HEISMAN** 20 secs | 2 minute rest

Repeat for 2 more sets

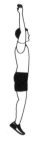 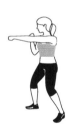 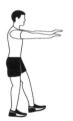 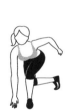 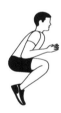 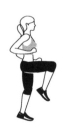 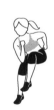

Perform each exercise as many times as possible within 20 seconds. Rest for 10 seconds then perform the next exercise again for 20 secs with a 10 sec rest in between exercises. Repeat until all 7 exercises have been completed.

Rest for 2 minutes then repeat the whole set two more times with a 2 minute rest in between.

Remember that these are high intensity workouts so try to push yourself to get as many repetitions of each exercise with the correct form within the 20 second period.

Burpees

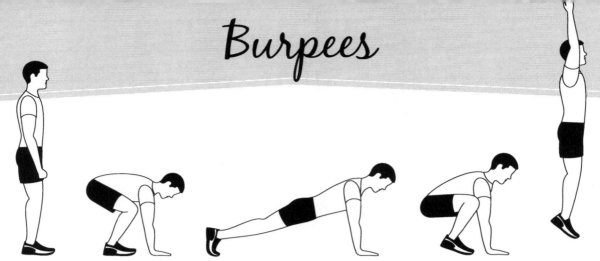

Stand with your feet shoulder-width apart, with your arms at your sides. Push your hips back, bend your knees, and lower your body into a squat before placing your hands on the floor directly in front of, and just inside, your feet. Jump your feet back to land in a plank position forming a straight line from head to toe with a straight back. Jump your feet back again so that they land just outside of your hands. Reach your arms over head and explosively jump up into the air. Land and immediately lower back into a squat for your next repetition.

Jab SQUATS

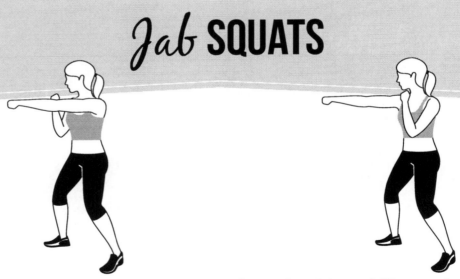

Start in a half squat position with your feet shoulder-width apart and knees slightly bent. Bring your arms up so the palms are facing the sides of your face. Clench your fists. Use sharp movements to lengthen your right arm in front in a punching motion then return to the starting position immediately punching out your left arm. Keep switching sides in a quick powerful motion.

Mummy KICKS

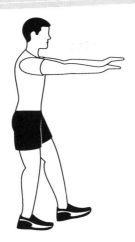 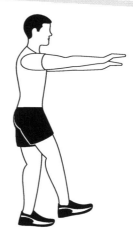

Begin by standing with your arms extended straight out in front. Perform light hop kicks with your feet while simultaneously criss-crossing your hands. Alternate the motion of your arms and hands as you swap between legs. Keep your core tight.

Side SKATER

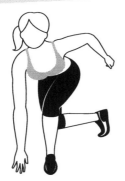 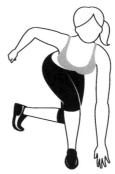

Start in a squat position with your left leg bent at the knee and your right arm parallel for balance. Your right leg is extended but still bent at the knee behind you. Jump sideways to the right, landing on your right leg. Bring your left leg behind you with your left arm extended and fingers touching the floor. Keep your back straight and your core engaged. Reverse direction by jumping to the left.

Tuck **JUMP**

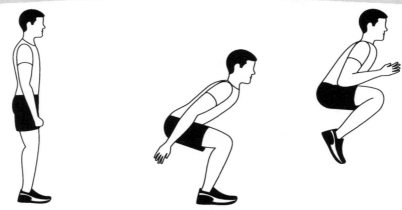

Begin in a standing position with knees slightly bent and arms at your sides. Bend your knees and lower your body quickly into a squat position, then explosively jump upwards bringing your knees up towards your chest.

Sprints

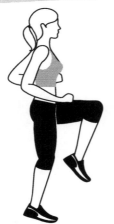 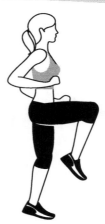

Standing with your feet shoulder-width apart, move your arms and torso as though you are running as fast as you can on the spot. Move feet and legs as little as possible avoiding twisting from side to side.

Heisman

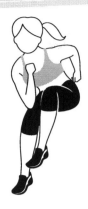 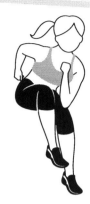

Begin by standing with feet shoulder-width apart and knees slightly bent. Jump onto your right foot while pulling your left knee up and towards the left shoulder. Next jump onto your left foot while pulling your right knee towards the right shoulder. Continue the movement in a quick motion, switching between legs.

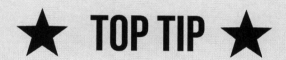

★ **TOP TIP** ★

Use a timer or stopwatch to precisely time each exercise and your rest time. There are many free apps available online. Try searching for 'tabata timer app'.

HiiT WORKOUT THREE

- Exercise 1: **SIT UPS** 20 secs | 10 secs rest
- Exercise 2: **BICYCLE CRUNCH** 20 secs | 10 secs rest
- Exercise 3: **MUMMY KICKS** 20 secs | 10 secs rest
- Exercise 4: **JAB SQUATS** 20 secs | 10 secs rest
- Exercise 5: **LATERALS** 20 secs | 10 secs rest
- Exercise 6: **MOUNTAIN CLIMBER** 20 secs | 10 sec rest
- Exercise 7: **TAP UP** 20 secs | 2 minute rest

Repeat for 2 more sets

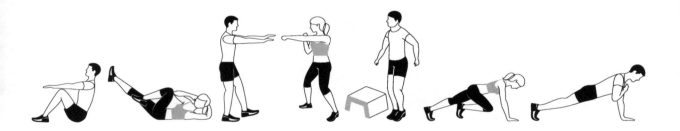

Perform each exercise as many times as possible within 20 seconds. Rest for 10 seconds then perform the next exercise again for 20 secs with a 10 sec rest in between exercises. Repeat until all 7 exercises have been completed.

Rest for 2 minutes then repeat the whole set two more times with a 2 minute rest in between.

Remember that these are high intensity workouts so try to push yourself to get as many repetitions of each exercise with the correct form within the 20 second period.

Sit UPS

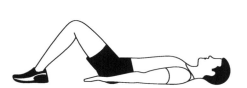 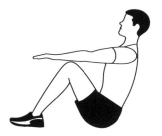

Lie on your back with your knees bent and your arms extended at your sides. and your feet flat on the floor. Engage your core and slowly curl your upper back off the floor towards your knees with your arms extended out. Roll back down to the starting position.

Bicycle CRUNCH

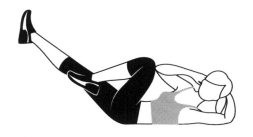 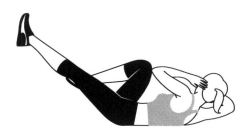

Lie face up and place your hands at the side of your head (do not pull on the back of your head). Make sure your core is tight and the small of your back is pushed hard against the floor. Lift your knees in toward your chest while lifting your shoulder blades off the floor. Rotate to the right, bringing the left elbow towards the right knee as you extend the other leg into the air. Switch sides, bringing the right elbow towards the left knee. Alternate each side in a pedaling motion..

Mummy KICKS

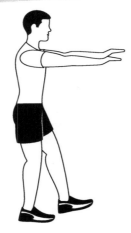 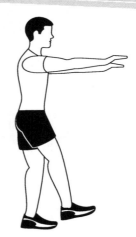

Begin by standing with your arms extended straight out in front. Perform light hop kicks with your feet while simultaneously criss-crossing your hands. Alternate the motion of your arms and hands as you swap between legs. Keep your core tight.

Jab SQUATS

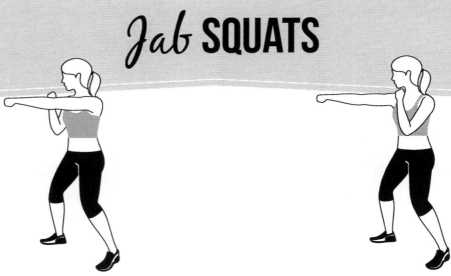

Start in a half squat position with your feet shoulder-width apart and knees slightly bent. Bring your arms up so the palms are facing the sides of your face. Clench your fists. Use sharp movements to lengthen your right arm in front in a punching motion then return to the starting position immediately punching out your left arm. Keep switching sides in a quick powerful motion.

Laterals

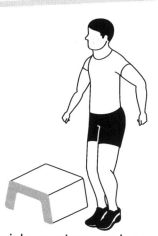 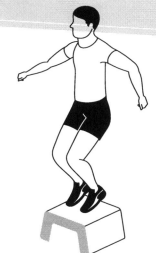

Stand beside a step or box. Position into a quarter squat then jump up and over to the right landing on the box with both feet landing together. Bring your knees high enough to ensure your feet clear the box. Jump over to the other side and repeat, this time jumping to the left.

Mountain CLIMBER

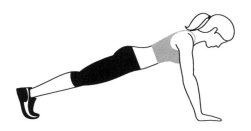 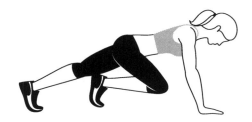

Begin in a pushup position, with your weight supported by your hands and toes. Flexing the knee and hip, bring one leg towards the corresponding arm. Explosively reverse the positions of your legs, extending the bent leg until the leg is straight and supported by the toe, and bringing the other foot up with the hip and knee flexed. Repeat in an alternating fashion.

Tap UPS

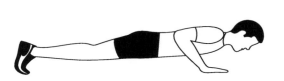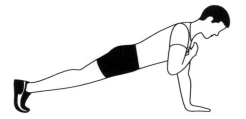

Begin in a pushup/plank position with your hands slightly wider than shoulder-width apart. Bend your elbows to lower your body to the floor just like a normal pushup. Pause, press back up to the starting position then tap one shoulder with the opposite side's hand. Repeat tapping the opposite shoulder.

★ TOP TIP ★

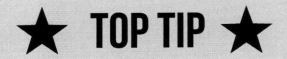

Work as hard as you can in each 30 sec burst. This is high intensity training so give maximum effort while maintaining correct form for each exercise.

- Exercise 1: **PRESS UPS** 20 secs | 10 secs rest
- Exercise 2: **SQUAT LUNGE** 20 secs | 10 secs rest
- Exercise 3: **STANDING STRAIGHT LEG BICYCLE** 20 secs | 10 secs rest
- Exercise 4: **TUCK JUMPS** 20 secs | 10 secs rest
- Exercise 5: **STANDING MOUNTAIN CLIMBERS** 20 secs | 10 secs rest
- Exercise 6: **BURPEES** 20 secs | 10 sec rest
- Exercise 6: **SCISSOR JUMPS** 20 secs | 2 minute rest

Repeat for 2 more sets

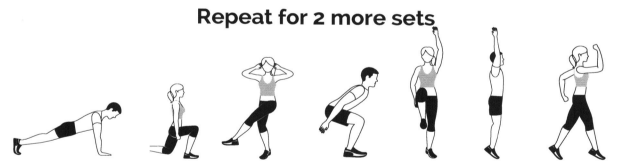

Perform each exercise as many times as possible within 30 seconds or hold for the desired length of time depending on the drill. Rest for 10 seconds then perform the next exercise again for 30 secs with a 10 sec rest in between exercises. Repeat until all 6 exercises have been completed.

Rest for 2 minutes then repeat the whole set two more times with a 2 minute rest in between.

Press UPS

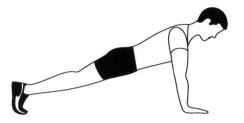

Begin in a high plank position with your hands shoulder-width apart. Lower your body ensuring you keep it aligned and look ahead to avoid strain in the neck. When your chest brushes the floor push back up. If you find this move difficult, start with your knees on the floor lowering only your upper torso.

Squat LUNGE

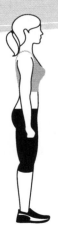 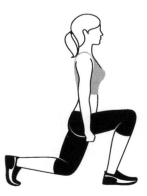

Stand upright with feet hip-width apart and arms at your sides. Take a controlled step forward with your right leg, keeping balance so that both knees are at 90 degree angles. Make sure your hips are low and back is straight. Push back with your right leg to the starting position. Repeat on left leg.

Standing Straight Leg BICYCLE

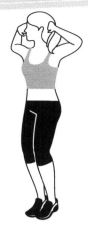 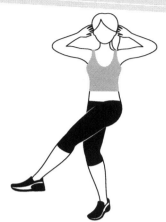

Begin by standing tall, hands touching the sides of your head but not clasped, feet shoulder-width apart. Opening your elbows wide, bring your right elbow down while simultaneously raising your left knee till they meet. Return to the starting position then repeat with left elbow to right knee. Opposite elbows go to opposite knees.

Tuck JUMP

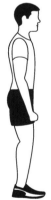 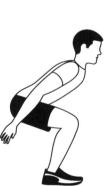 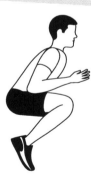

Begin in a standing position with knees slightly bent and arms at your sides. Bend your knees and lower your body quickly into a squat position, then explosively jump upwards bringing your knees up towards your chest.

Standing MOUNTAIN CLIMBER

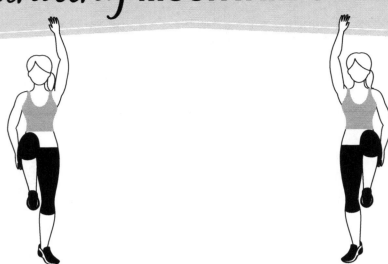

Begin by standing with feet shoulder-width apart and arms by your side. Bring your left knee up to waist level while extending your right arm to the sky. Return to the starting position then repeat this time raising your right knee and left arm. Keep alternating sides in a climbing motion.

Burpees

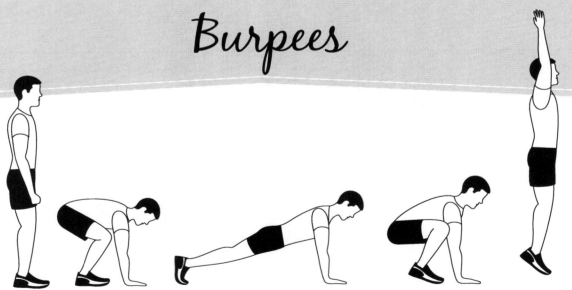

Lie on your back and extend your arms out to the side. Raise your knees and feet so they create a 90-degree angle. Contract your abdominals and exhale as you lift your hips off the floor. Your knees will move toward your head. Try to keep your knees at a right angle. Inhale and slowly lower.

Scissor JUMPS

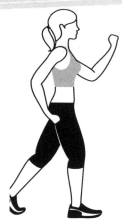 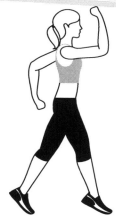

Begin by standing with right foot approx. 2 feet in front of left. Right arm should be extended behind you and left arm in front of you with elbows bent as if in a running position. Quickly jump up while switching arm and leg positions while in the air, landing with left foot in front of right foot and right arm in front of your body, left arm behind you. Continue alternating arms and legs while jumping.

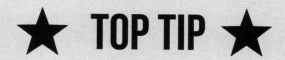

Keep your core tight! By keeping your abdominal area firm, not only are you working the ab muscles but also keeping a strong mid-section which is vital for balance and control.

Straight Leg Calf STRETCH

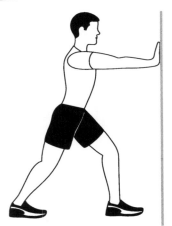 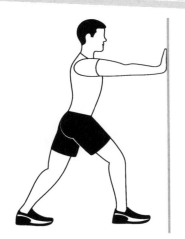

Place both hands on a wall with arms extended. Lean against the wall with right leg bent forward and left leg extended behind with knee straight and feet positioned directly forward. Push rear heal to floor and move hips slightly forward holding the stretch for 10 secs. Repeat with opposite leg.

Shoulder STRETCH

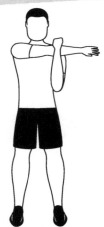 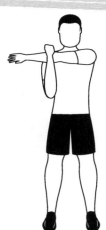

The right arm is placed over the left shoulder. Position the wrist on your left arm to the elbow of your right arm gently pushing towards the shoulder. Swap shoulders.

Standing Quadricep STRETCH

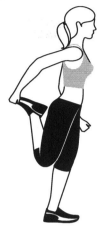 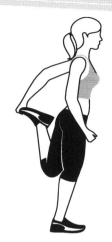

Begin by standing with your feet hip-width apart. Bend your right leg backwards grasping the right foot to bring your heel toward your buttocks. Hold for 5-10 secs then repeat for left leg. Use your opposite arm to balance if need be.

Lower Back STRETCH

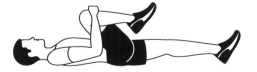 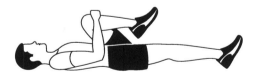

Begin by lying flat on your back with toes pointed upward. Slowly bend your right knee and pull your leg up to you chest, wrapping your arms around your thigh and hands clasped around the knee or shin. Gently pull the knee towards your chest and hold for 10 secs. Repeat on left leg.

Cat Cow STRETCH

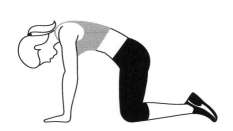 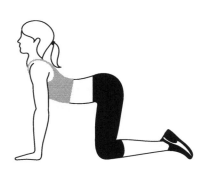

Begin with your hands and knees on the floor. Exhale while rounding your spine up towards the ceiling, pulling your belly button up towards your spine, and engaging your core. Inhale while arching your back and letting your tummy relax.

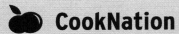 CookNation

Other COOKNATION TITLES

If you enjoyed **The** *Skinny* **15 Minute Meals &** *HIIT* **Workout Plan** you may also be interested in other *Skinny* titles in the CookNation series.

Visit **www.bellmackenzie.com** to browse the full catalogue.